Everyday Yoga Day

35 Poses for the whole month, for beginners to advanced 2023

Stefan Becker

ISBN-13: 9798375338149
ISBN-10: 1477123456

Cover design by: Art Painter
Library of Congress Control Number: 2018675309
Printed in the United States of America

Contents

Everyday Yoga Day

35 Poses for the whole month, for beginners to advanced

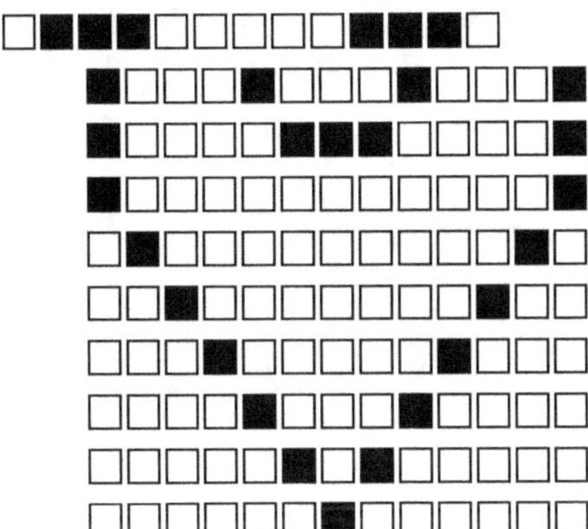

"Unleash the power of yoga with our comprehensive guide, featuring 35 dynamic poses for the entire month. Suitable for both beginners and advanced practitioners, this book will take you on a journey of physical and mental transformation. Start each day with a new pose and discover the benefits of increased flexibility, strength, and balance. From the grounding mountain pose to the energizing warrior series, this guide is your ultimate tool for achieving a stronger, more peaceful body and mind. Whether you're looking to improve your athletic performance or simply seeking a daily dose of tranquility, this book has something for everyone."

Bow Pose

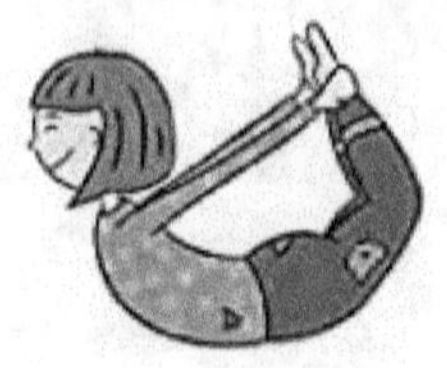

Bow Pose

Bow Pose, also known as Dhanurasana, is a dynamic backbend yoga pose that is considered to be an intermediate level pose. It is said to be beneficial for strengthening the back and arm muscles, and for stretching the chest, abdominal muscles and hips.

To come into the pose, begin by lying on your stomach with your arms alongside your body. Bend your knees and reach back to grab the inside of your ankles. As you inhale, lift your head and chest off the ground, and use the strength of your back muscles to lift your legs off the ground. Keep your gaze forward and your breath steady.

It's important to engage your core, lift your chest and keep your breath steady. It's also important to come out of the pose slowly and with mindful movements.

Bow Pose is considered to be a very beneficial pose for strengthening the back muscles and stretching the chest and abdominal muscles. Additionally, it helps to open the hips and improve flexibility of the spine. It's also a good pose to practice before and after other backbends.

Butterfly Pose

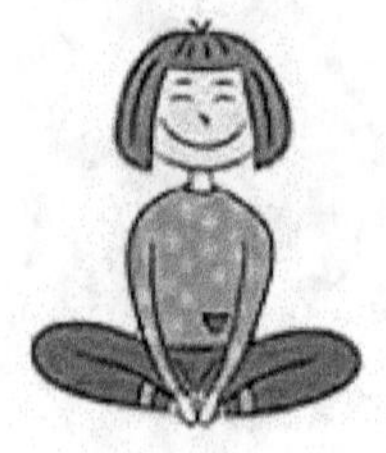

Butterfly Pose

Butterfly Pose, also known as Baddha Konasana, is a seated yoga pose that is considered to be a beginner level pose. It is said to be beneficial for the hips, inner thighs, and lower back, as well as for improving digestion and reducing stress.

To come into the pose, begin by sitting on the floor with your legs extended out in front of you. Bend your knees and bring the soles of your feet together, so that the heels are close to your body. Hold onto your feet with your hands and gently press your knees down towards the floor. Sit up tall, with your spine straight and your shoulders relaxed. You can use a block or cushion to sit on if your hips are not able to touch the floor comfortably.

It's important to keep the spine tall and to engage the thigh muscles to protect the knee joints. You can use a block or cushion to sit on

if your hips are not able to touch the floor comfortably. It's also important to come out of the pose slowly and with mindful movements.

Butterfly pose is considered to be a very beneficial pose for the hip, inner thigh and lower back muscles. It's also a good pose for those who spend a lot of time sitting, as it helps to stretch out the hips and inner thigh muscles. It's also a good pose to practice before seated forward bends, as it helps to prepare the body. It's also good for releasing tension in the groins and lower back.

Camel Pose

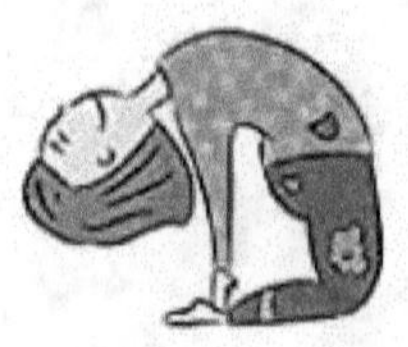

Camel Pose

Camel Pose, also known as Ustrasana, is a yoga pose that opens the chest and strengthens the back muscles. It is considered to be an intermediate level pose, as it requires a certain level of flexibility and strength in the back and legs.

To come into the pose, begin on your knees with your knees hip-width apart and your thighs perpendicular to the floor. Place your hands on your lower back with your fingers pointing down. As you inhale, lift your chest and press your hips forward, reaching back to grab your heels. Keep your head in a neutral position, looking straight ahead.

Camel Pose is a great way to open the chest and improve the flexibility of the spine. It also helps to strengthen the back muscles and improve posture. It's a great pose

to practice when you are feeling stiff or tight in the chest
or when you want to improve your breathing.

It's important to keep the core engaged and the legs strong, to keep the neck and spine in a neutral position and avoid straining the lower back. This pose is not recommended for people with lower back or neck injuries or high blood pressure. It's also important to use props or have a teacher's assistance when practicing this pose.

Cat Pose

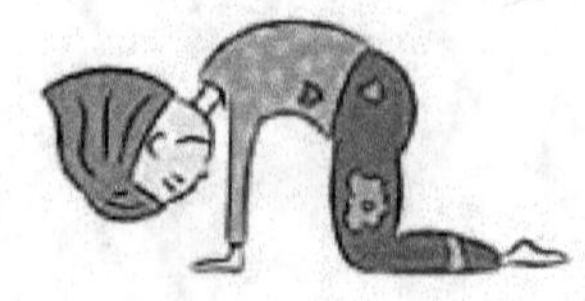

Cat Pose

Cat Pose, also known as Marjaryasana, is a yoga pose that is often used as a counter pose to Cow Pose. It is a gentle pose that helps to stretch the spine and release tension in the back and neck. It is considered to be a beginner level pose.

To come into the pose, begin on your hands and knees with your wrists directly under your shoulders and your knees directly under your hips. As you exhale, round your spine towards the ceiling, tucking your chin into your chest and bringing your tailbone towards your knees. Your arms should be straight and your shoulders relaxed.

Cat Pose is a great way to stretch the spine and release tension in the back and neck. It also helps to strengthen the back muscles and improve posture. It's a great pose to practice

when you are feeling stiff or tight in the back or when you want
to warm up the spine before practicing other yoga poses.

It's important to keep the shoulders relaxed and away from the
ears, to keep the wrists in line with the shoulders and keep the core
engaged. Keep the gaze to the navel and avoid straining the neck.
Some people may feel discomfort in the lower back, if this is the
case, it's important to move gently and avoid over-arching the back.

Chair Pose

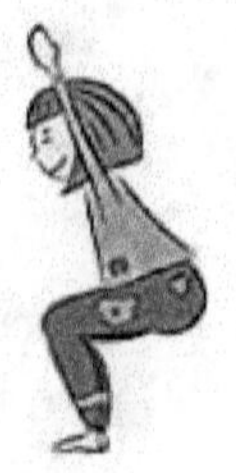

Chair Pose

Chair Pose, also known as Utkatasana, is a standing yoga pose that is known for strengthening the legs and core, as well as improving balance and focus.

To come into the pose, begin by standing in Mountain Pose (Tadasana) with your feet together and your arms at your sides. Ground down through the four corners of your feet and engage your thigh muscles to lift the kneecaps. Draw the tailbone down towards the floor and lengthen the spine upward, creating a sense of lengthening through the crown of the head. Bring your shoulder blades down and back, and bend your knees, bringing your thighs as close to parallel with the floor as possible. Bring your arms up to the sides of your body, parallel with the floor, with the palms facing forward. Keep your gaze forward and breathe deeply. Hold the pose for several breaths.

As you hold the pose, try to engage your core and press

your hips down and back, as if you were sitting back into an invisible chair. This will help to strengthen the legs, glutes and core. The pose also stretches the spine and chest, opens the shoulders and improves balance and focus.

Child Pose

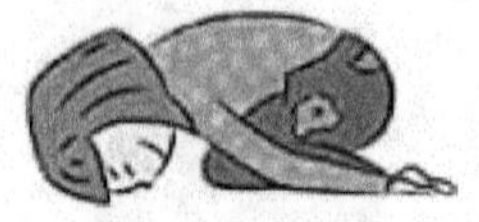

Child Pose

Child's Pose, also known as Balasana, is a restorative and calming yoga pose that is considered to be a beginner level pose. It is said to be beneficial for stretching the hips, thighs, and ankles, and for relieving stress and tension in the back.

To come into the pose, begin by kneeling on the floor with your knees hip-width apart and your big toes touching. Sit back on your heels and then lean forward, stretching your arms out in front of you. Rest your forehead on the ground and relax your entire body. You can also bring your arms back alongside your body, with your palms facing up. Keep your breath steady and your gaze soft.

It's important to keep your breath steady and to come out of the pose slowly and with mindful movements.

Child's Pose is considered to be a very beneficial pose for stretching the hips, thighs, and ankles. Additionally, it helps to release tension in the back and shoulders, and also helps to improve digestion. It's also a great pose to practice before and after backbends, and also a good pose for relaxation.

Cobra Pose

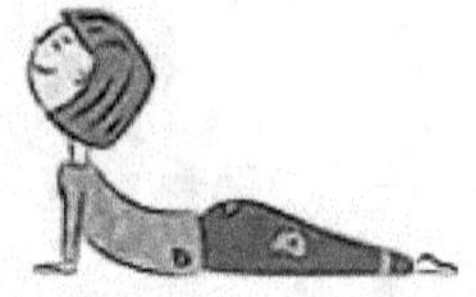

Cobra Pose

Cobra Pose, also known as Bhujangasana, is a strengthening and energizing yoga pose that is considered to be a beginner level pose. It is said to be beneficial for strengthening the back muscles and for opening the chest and shoulders.

To come into the pose, begin by lying on your stomach with your hands placed beside your chest, fingers pointing forward. As you inhale, press into your hands and lift your chest off the ground. Keep your elbows close to your body and your shoulders relaxed. Keep your gaze forward and your breath steady.

It's important to engage your back muscles and keep your elbows close to your body. It's also important to come out of the pose slowly and with mindful movements.

Cobra Pose is considered to be a very beneficial pose for strengthening the back muscles and opening the chest and shoulders. Additionally, it helps to improve posture and to relieve stress and tension in the back. It's also a good pose to practice before and after other backbends.

Corpse Pose

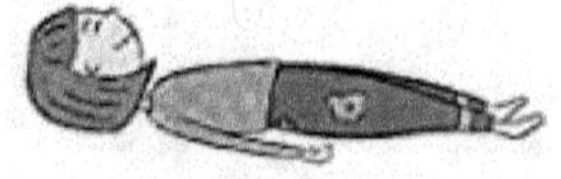

Corpse Pose

Corpse Pose, also known as Savasana, is a relaxation pose that is often practiced at the end of a yoga session. The pose is designed to relax the body, quiet the mind, and promote a sense of inner stillness and calm.

To come into the pose, begin by lying on your back with your feet hip-width apart and your arms by your sides. Let your feet fall open and your arms relax, away from the body. Close your eyes and take a deep breath in through your nose, and then exhale through your mouth.

As you lie in the pose, focus on relaxing each part of your body, starting with your toes and working your way up to the top of your head. Release any tension or tightness that you may be holding in your body.

Breathe deeply and slowly, allowing your breath to become slow and even. Let go of any thoughts or distractions, and allow yourself to sink into a state of deep relaxation.

Stay in the pose for as long as you like, ideally for at least 5-10 minutes. When you're ready to come out of the pose, take a deep breath in and then slowly roll onto your right side. Pause for a moment and then use your hands to push yourself up to a seated position.

Corpse pose is considered to be one of the most important yoga poses as it helps to calm the mind, release tension in the body, and promote a sense of inner peace and tranquility. Additionally, it is said to be beneficial for reducing stress, fatigue, and tension headaches.

Cow Pose

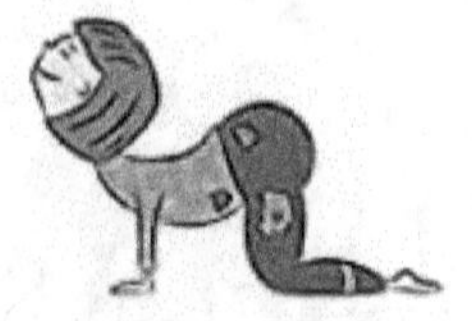

Cow Pose

Cow Pose, also known as Bitilasana, is a yoga pose that is often used as a counter pose to Cat Pose. It is a gentle pose that helps to stretch the spine and open the chest. It is considered to be a beginner level pose.

To come into the pose, begin on your hands and knees with your wrists directly under your shoulders and your knees directly under your hips. As you inhale, lift your sitting bones and chest towards the ceiling, allowing your belly to sink towards the floor. Arch your back and lift your head, looking up towards the ceiling. Your arms should be straight and your shoulders relaxed.

Cow Pose is a great way to stretch the spine and open the chest. It also helps to strengthen the back muscles and improve posture. It's a great pose to practice when you

are feeling stiff or tight in the back or when you want to
warm up the spine before practicing other yoga poses.

It's important to keep the shoulders relaxed and away from the
ears, to keep the wrists in line with the shoulders and keep the core
engaged. Keep the gaze forward and avoid straining the neck.
Some people may feel discomfort in the lower back, if this is the
case, it's important to move gently and avoid over-arching the back.

Downward Facing Dog

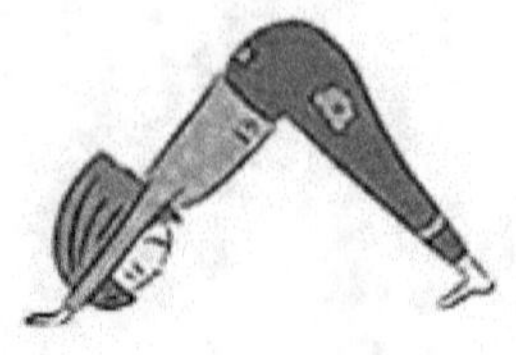

Downward Facing Pose

Downward Facing Dog, also known as Adho Mukha Svanasana, is a well-known and widely practiced yoga pose that is known for its ability to stretch the entire body, particularly the spine, hamstrings, calves, and hands. It is also considered a mild inversion and can help to improve circulation and relieve stress.

To come into the pose, begin on your hands and knees with your wrists directly under your shoulders and your knees directly under your hips. As you exhale, lift your hips up and back, straightening your arms and legs and coming into an inverted "V" shape. Press your hands and feet into the ground and lengthen through your spine. Keep your gaze towards your navel or towards your knees. Hold the pose for several deep breaths.

It is a great pose to stretch out the whole body, particularly the spine, hamstrings, calves, and hands. It also provides a great release for the neck and shoulders and helps to calm the mind. It is also a great way to improve circulation and relieve stress.

It's important to keep the hands and feet pressing firmly into the ground, and lengthening the spine and tailbone to the ceiling. Also, make sure to keep your heels towards the ground and engage the leg muscles, and avoid rounding the shoulders, and keep the neck relaxed by keeping gaze at navel or towards the knees. It can be modified by using a wall or a chair if you have difficulty keeping your heels on the ground.

Easy Pose

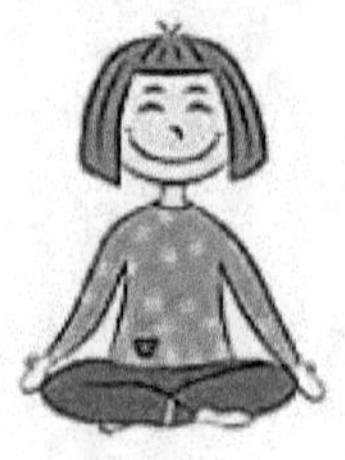

Easy Pose

Easy Pose, also known as Sukhasana, is a yoga pose that is considered to be a basic seated posture, often used for meditation and pranayama (breathing exercises). It is considered to be a beginner level pose, as it is relatively easy to perform.

To come into the pose, begin by sitting on the floor with your legs crossed, with the right foot on top of the left thigh and the left foot on top of the right thigh. You can also bring the feet together and sit on the heels if you are more flexible. Sit up tall, with your spine straight and your shoulders relaxed. Place your hands on your knees or in a mudra (hand gesture) of your choice.

Easy Pose is said to be beneficial for the mind and body, as it helps to improve posture and balance, increase flexibility in the hips, and calm the mind and nervous system. It's also said to be beneficial for people with lower back pain, as it helps to stretch and strengthen the lower back muscles.

Easy Pose is a comfortable and accessible position that can be practiced by people of all ages and levels of flexibility. It's also a good position to use as a base for other meditative poses, such as the Lotus Pose.

Extended Corpse Pose

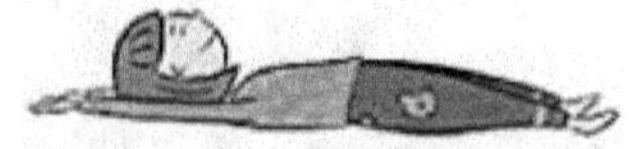

Extended Corpse Pose

Extended Corpse Pose, also known as Supta Savasana, is a variation of the traditional Corpse Pose (Savasana) that involves extending the arms out to the sides in a T-shape. This variation allows for an even deeper release of tension in the shoulders and chest, and can be especially helpful for those experiencing stress or anxiety.

To come into the pose, begin by lying on your back with your feet hip-width apart and your arms by your sides. Let your feet fall open and your arms relax, away from the body. Close your eyes and take a deep breath in through your nose, and then exhale through your mouth.

As you exhale, extend your arms out to the sides in a T-shape, with your palms facing up. Allow your shoulders to relax down and away from your ears, and let your chest expand with each breath.

As you inhale, focus on lengthening through your spine, and as you exhale, release any tension or tightness in your body.

Stay in the pose for as long as you like, ideally for at least 5-10 minutes. When you're ready to come out of the pose, take a deep breath in and then slowly roll onto your right side. Pause for a moment and then use your hands to push yourself up to a seated position.

This variation of corpse pose is considered to be a more advanced version of the traditional pose, and it is said to be beneficial for reducing stress, fatigue, and tension headaches. Additionally, it can help to improve the flexibility of the shoulder and chest, and promote a sense of inner peace and tranquility.

Extended Mountain Pose

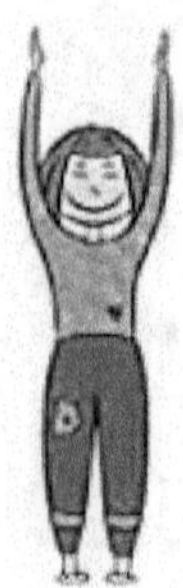

Extendend Mountain Pose

Extended Mountain Pose, also known as Utthita Tadasana, is a variation of the basic Mountain Pose (Tadasana) in which the arms are raised above the head. It is considered a beginner-intermediate level pose and is known for helping to improve posture, balance, and core strength.

To come into the pose, begin by standing in Mountain Pose (Tadasana) with your feet together and your arms at your sides. Ground down through the four corners of your feet and engage your thigh muscles to lift the kneecaps. Draw the tailbone down towards the floor and lengthen the spine upward, creating a sense of lengthening through the crown of the head. Bring your shoulder blades down and back, and raise your arms above your head, with the palms facing each other. Keep your gaze forward and breathe deeply. Hold the pose for several breaths.

It is a great pose for stretching the entire body, especially the spine and arms, and can help to improve focus and concentration. It also strengthens the legs, feet and core.

Five-Pointed Star Pose

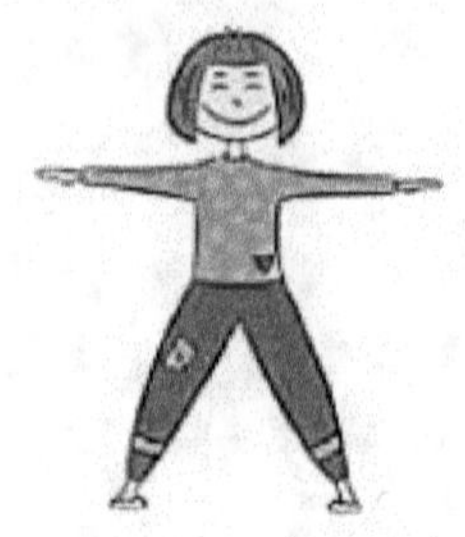

Five-Pointed Star Pose

Five-Pointed Star Pose, also known as Utthita Tadasana with Extended Arms, is a variation of the basic Mountain Pose (Tadasana) with the arms extended out to the sides and one leg lifted up. It is considered an intermediate-level pose and is known for helping to improve balance, focus and core strength.

To come into the pose, begin by standing in Mountain Pose (Tadasana) with your feet together and your arms at your sides. Ground down through the four corners of your feet and engage your thigh muscles to lift the kneecaps. Draw the tailbone down towards the floor and lengthen the spine upward, creating a sense of lengthening through the crown of the head. Bring your shoulder blades down and back, and extend your arms out to the sides at shoulder level, with the palms facing forward. Then, shift your weight to one foot and lift the other leg off the ground, keeping the knee straight. Keep your gaze forward and breathe deeply. Hold the pose for several breaths before switching sides.

It is a challenging balance pose that requires concentration, focus, and core stability. It also strengthens the legs, feet and core, as well as improves balance and focus.

Garland Pose

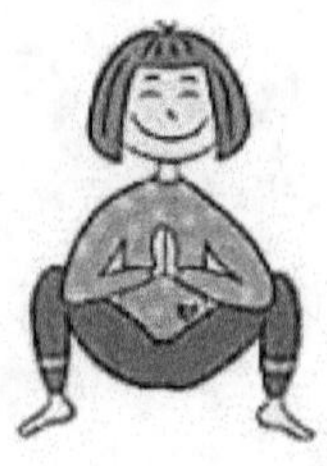

Garland Pose

Garland Pose, also known as Malasana, is a deep squatting
yoga pose that is considered to be an intermediate level pose.
It is said to be beneficial for the hips, thighs, and lower back,
as well as for improving digestion and reducing stress.

To come into the pose, begin by standing with your feet
wider than hip-width apart. Turn your toes out to the
sides, and bend your knees to lower your hips towards the
floor. Bring your hands together in front of your heart in
a prayer position. As you lower your hips, bring your torso
forward and rest your elbows on the inside of your knees.
Keep your spine straight and your shoulders relaxed.

It's important to keep the spine tall and to engage the thigh muscles
to protect the knee joints. You can use a block or cushion to sit on

if your hips are not able to touch the floor comfortably. It's also important to come out of the pose slowly and with mindful movements.

Garland Pose is considered to be a very beneficial pose for the hip, thigh, and lower back muscles. It's also a good pose for those who spend a lot of time sitting, as it helps to stretch out the hips and thigh muscles. It's also a good pose to practice before seated forward bends, as it helps to prepare the body. Additionally, it helps to open the hips, groin and lower back, and also helps to release tension in the lower back.

Happy Baby Pose

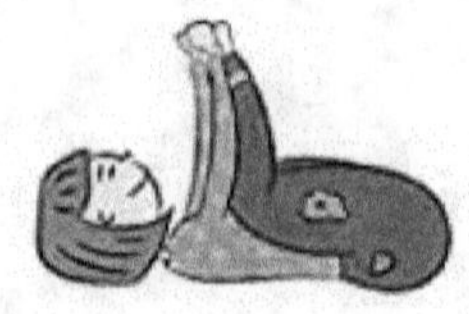

Happy Baby Pose

Happy Baby Pose, also known as Ananda Balasana,
is a playful and restorative yoga pose that is considered
to be a beginner level pose. It is said to be beneficial
for opening the hips, lower back, and inner groins.

To come into the pose, begin by lying on your back with your
knees bent and your feet flat on the floor. Bring your knees
towards your armpits, and then reach back and grab the outer
edges of your feet with your hands. Keep your feet flexed and
your knees pointing towards the ceiling. Gently pull your knees
down towards the floor, while keeping your low back pressed into
the ground. Keep your breath steady and your gaze soft.

It's important to keep your low back pressed into the ground,
and to keep your breath steady. It's also important to come

out of the pose slowly and with mindful movements.

Happy Baby Pose is considered to be a very beneficial pose for opening the hips and lower back. Additionally, it helps to release tension in the inner groins, and also helps to improve digestion. It's also a great pose to practice before deep hip openers and twists.

Hero Pose

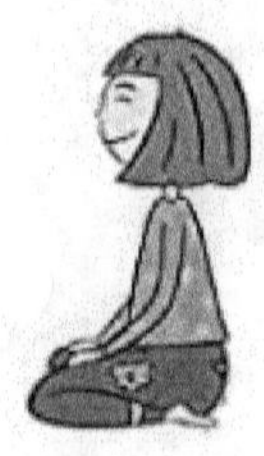

Hero Pose

Hero Pose, also known as Virasana, is a kneeling yoga pose that is considered to be an intermediate level pose. It is said to be beneficial for the knees, thighs, and lower back, as well as for improving digestion and reducing stress.

To come into the pose, begin by kneeling on the floor with your knees together and your big toes touching. Lower your hips back towards your heels and sit down on the floor. You can use a block or cushion to sit on if your hips are not able to touch the floor comfortably. Sit up tall, with your spine straight and your shoulders relaxed. Place your hands on your knees or in a mudra (hand gesture) of your choice.

It's important to keep the spine tall and to engage the thigh muscles to protect the knee joints. You can use a block or cushion to sit on

if your hips are not able to touch the floor comfortably. It's also important to come out of the pose slowly and with mindful movements.

Hero Pose is considered to be a very beneficial pose for the knee and thigh muscles, and also for the digestion and stress. It's also a good pose for those who spend a lot of time sitting, as it helps to stretch out the hips and strengthen the thigh muscles. It's also a good pose to practice before seated forward bends, as it helps to prepare the body.

Knee to Chest Pose

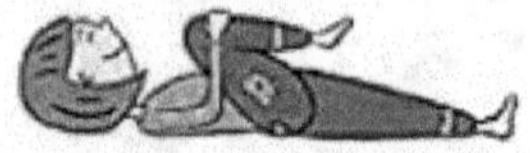

Knee to chest Pose

Knee to Chest Pose, also known as Apanasana, is a gentle yoga pose that is considered to be a beginner level pose. It is said to be beneficial for stretching the lower back and for relieving stress and tension in the back.

To come into the pose, begin by lying on your back with your knees bent and your feet on the ground. As you inhale, bring one knee in towards your chest and hold it with your hands. Keep your other foot on the ground. As you exhale, release the knee and repeat with the other leg. Keep your gaze forward and your breath steady.

It's important to keep your lower back relaxed and to come in and out of the pose slowly and with mindful movements.

Knee to Chest Pose is considered to be a very beneficial pose for stretching the lower back and for relieving stress and tension in the back. Additionally, it helps to improve flexibility and mobility in the hips, legs and back. It's also a good pose to practice before and after other backbends or forward folds.

Knees to Chest-Chin Pose

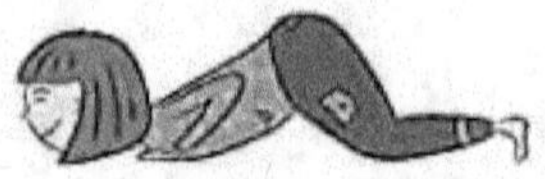

Knees to Chest-Chin Pose

Knees-Chest-Chin Pose, also known as Apanasana
with Chin Lock, is an advanced variation of the Knee to
Chest Pose. This pose is designed to increase the stretch
on the lower back and to strengthen the core muscles.

To come into the pose, begin by lying on your back with your knees
bent and your feet on the ground. As you inhale, bring your knees in
towards your chest and hold them with your hands. As you exhale,
tuck your chin in towards your chest, keeping your gaze forward.

As you inhale, lift your head and shoulders off the ground, bringing
your chest closer to your knees. Exhale and release the pose.

It's important to practice this pose under the guidance of an

experienced teacher, as it can be quite challenging for beginners.
It's also important to keep the lower back relaxed and to come
in and out of the pose slowly and with mindful movements.

75

Knees-Chest-Chin Pose is considered to be beneficial
for stretching the lower back, strengthening the core
muscles, and improving flexibility and mobility in the hips,
legs and back. Additionally, it is said to be beneficial
for relieving stress and tension in the back.

Legs up the Wall Pose

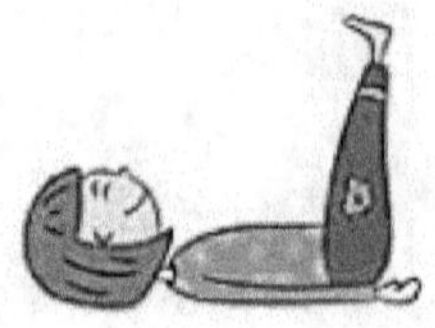

Legs up the Wall Pose

Leg Up the Wall Pose, also known as Viparita Karani, is a restorative yoga pose that is considered to be a beginner level pose. It is said to be beneficial for relieving stress, reducing fatigue, and improving circulation.

To come into the pose, begin by sitting on the floor with one hip against a wall. Then, swing your legs up onto the wall and lie down on your back. Your hips should be close to the wall, and your legs should be straight up against the wall. You can place a pillow or folded blanket under your hips for comfort. Allow your arms to rest at your sides, with your palms facing up. Close your eyes and breathe deeply, allowing your body to relax.

It's important to keep your spine straight and your neck relaxed, and keep your breath steady. It's also important to come out of the pose slowly and with mindful movements.

Leg Up the Wall pose is considered to be a very beneficial pose for relieving stress and reducing fatigue. It's also a good pose for those who spend a lot of time sitting or standing, as it helps to improve circulation. Additionally, it helps to release tension in the lower back and legs, and also helps to improve digestion.

Lotus Pose

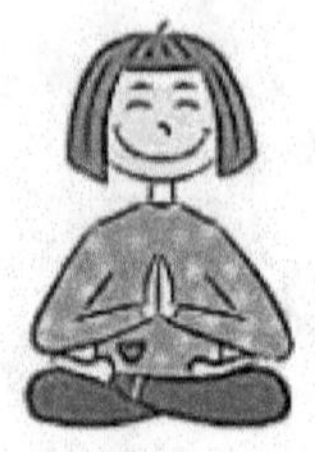

Lotus Pose

Lotus Pose, also known as Padmasana, is a yoga pose that is considered to be one of the most important and traditional seated meditation postures in yoga. It is considered to be an advanced level pose, as it requires a good level of flexibility and balance to perform.

To come into the pose, begin by sitting on the floor with your legs stretched out in front of you. Bend your right knee and bring the right foot to rest on the left thigh. Then, bend the left knee and bring the left foot to rest on the right thigh, with the soles of the feet facing up. Keep your back straight and your hands on your knees or in a mudra (hand gesture) of your choice.

Lotus Pose is said to be beneficial for the mind and body, as it helps to improve posture and balance, increase flexibility in the hips and knees, and calm the mind and nervous system.

It's also said to be beneficial for people with asthma, as
it helps to open the lungs and improve breathing.

It's important to practice Lotus Pose with a qualified teacher,
as it can be difficult to perform correctly without proper guidance.
Also, it's important to be mindful of the knees and hips, which
can be easily strained if the pose is done incorrectly. It's not
recommended for people with knee, hip or back injuries, or for those
who have not yet built up the necessary flexibility. It's also not
recommend to hold this pose for long periods of time if you are
not comfortable or prepared, as it may cause discomfort or pain.

Low Boat Pose

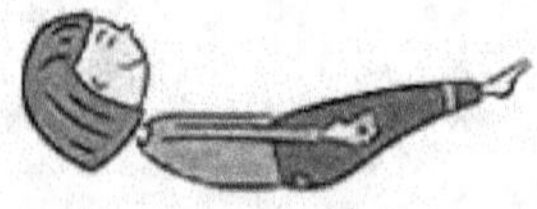

Low Boat Pose

Low Boat Pose, also known as Navasana, is a yoga pose that strengthens the core and improves balance and stability. It is considered an intermediate-level pose.

To come into the pose, sit on the mat with your knees bent and your feet flat on the floor. Place your hands behind your knees and lean back slightly, lifting your feet off the floor and balancing on your sit bones. Begin to straighten your legs, keeping them together, and lift your feet so that your shins are parallel to the floor. Reach your arms forward, parallel to the floor, with your palms facing each other. Keep your gaze forward and breathe deeply. Hold the pose for several breaths.

Low boat pose is a great way to strengthen the core, especially the rectus abdominis, obliques and the transverse abdominis muscles. It also helps to improve balance, focus, and stability. It also helps to build strength and flexibility in the legs and hips. It's an excellent pose for those looking to improve their balance and core strength.

It's important to keep the core engaged and avoid collapsing in the lower back, also to keep the legs parallel to the floor and the arms parallel to the floor. Keep the gaze forward and avoid straining the neck. You can make the pose more challenging by lifting the hands up and reaching forward or by straightening the legs more. If you have any lower back pain or injury, it's best to avoid this pose or to perform it with caution and under the guidance of a qualified instructor.

Lunge Pose

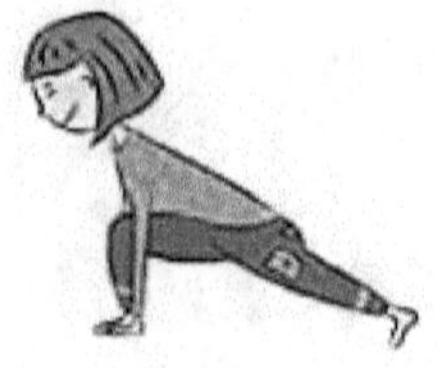

Lunge Post

Lunge Pose, also known as Anjaneyasana, is a yoga
pose that is known for stretching the hips, thighs, and
psoas muscle, as well as strengthening the legs and core.
It is considered an intermediate-level pose.

To come into the pose, begin in a standing position, then take a
large step forward with your left foot, placing your foot between
your hands. Your right knee should be pointing straight down
towards the ground, with your thigh parallel to the floor. Your
left knee should be bent at a 90-degree angle, with your thigh
perpendicular to the floor. Bring your hands to your hips and lift
your chest, then either bring your hands to your heart or reach your
arms up towards the ceiling. Keep your gaze forward and breathe
deeply. Hold the pose for several breaths before switching sides.

It is a great pose to stretch the hips, thighs and psoas muscle, as well as strengthening the legs and core. It also helps to open the chest and shoulders, while also helping to improve balance, focus, and stability. It also helps to build strength and flexibility in the legs and hips, and is great for stretching the front of the body.

It's important to keep the front knee behind the ankle and not to let it move forward past the toes, also to keep the back leg straight and engaged and to keep the tailbone down and engage the core. Keep your front knee at a 90-degree angle, and keep both legs in a straight line with the front knee. Also, make sure to keep your chest lifted and avoid collapsing in the front hip.

Mountain Pose Arms Out

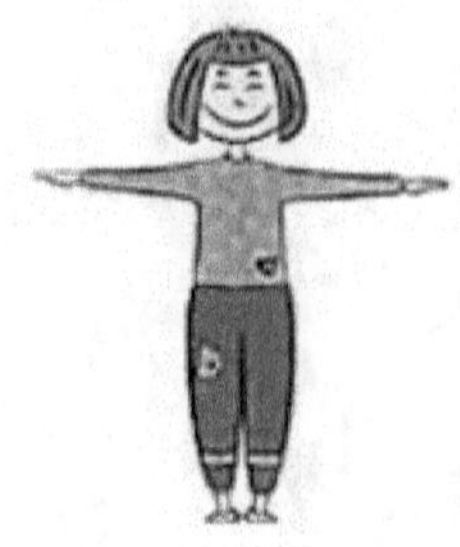

Mountain Pose Arms Out

Mountain Pose with Arms Out, also known as Tadasana with Extended Arms, is a variation of the basic Mountain Pose (Tadasana) in which the arms are extended out to the sides at shoulder level. It is considered a beginner-level pose and is known for helping to improve posture, balance, and core strength.

To come into the pose, begin by standing in Mountain Pose (Tadasana) with your feet together and your arms at your sides. Ground down through the four corners of your feet and engage your thigh muscles to lift the kneecaps. Draw the tailbone down towards the floor and lengthen the spine upward, creating a sense of lengthening through the crown of the head. Bring your shoulder blades down and back, and extend your arms out to the sides at shoulder level, with the palms facing forward. Keep your gaze forward and breathe deeply. Hold the pose for several breaths.

This variation of the Tadasana helps to open up the chest

and shoulders, and also strengthens the legs, feet and core.
It will also help with balance, focus and grounding.

95

Mountain Pose

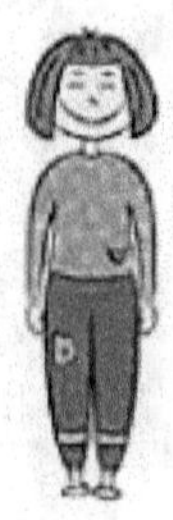

Mountain Pose

Mountain Pose, also known as Tadasana, is a standing yoga pose that serves as the foundation for many other yoga poses. It is considered a beginner-level pose and is known for helping to improve posture and balance.

To come into the pose, begin by standing with your feet together and your arms at your sides. Ground down through the four corners of your feet and engage your thigh muscles to lift the kneecaps. Draw the tailbone down towards the floor and lengthen the spine upward, creating a sense of lengthening through the crown of the head. Bring your shoulder blades down and back, and release your arms down by your sides, with the palms facing forward. Keep your gaze forward and breathe deeply. Hold the pose for several breaths.

It is the starting point of many yoga sequences, and can be used as a way to center and ground oneself before moving on to more challenging poses. It will help with developing balance, focus and grounding.

Plank Pose

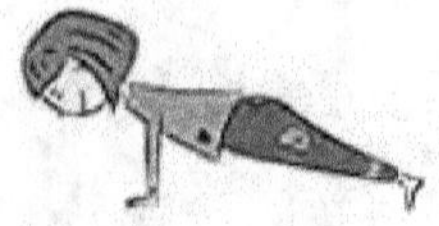

Plank Pose

Plank Pose, also known as *Kumbhakasana*, is a strengthening yoga pose that is considered to be a beginner to intermediate level pose. It is said to be beneficial for strengthening the core, arms, and shoulders and for toning the entire body.

To come into the pose, begin in a push-up position with your hands placed shoulder-width apart, your fingers pointing forward and your wrists under your shoulders. Keep your core engaged and your body straight, with your feet together. Keep your gaze forward and your breath steady.

It's important to engage your core and to keep your body in a straight line. It's also important to come out of the pose slowly and with mindful movements.

Plank Pose is considered to be a very beneficial pose for strengthening the core, arms, and shoulders and for toning the entire body. Additionally, it helps to improve posture, balance and stability. It's also a good pose to practice before and after other arm balances and inversions.

Plow Pose

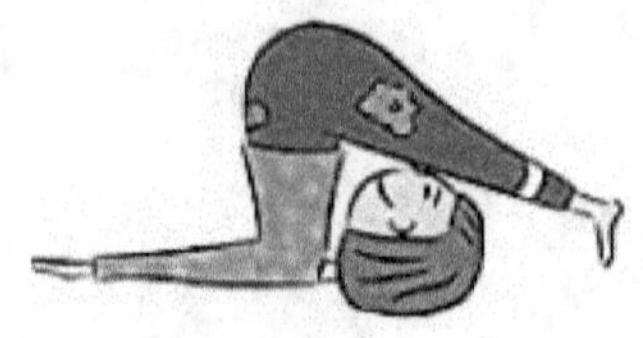

Plow Pose

Plow Pose, also known as Halasana, is a yoga pose that is said to have a number of benefits for the body, including stretching the spine, shoulders, and neck, as well as strengthening the core and legs. This pose is considered an intermediate level pose, as it requires a good level of flexibility and core strength to perform.

To come into the pose, lie on your back and lift your legs up towards the ceiling. Use your hands to support your lower back as you bring your legs over your head, attempting to touch your toes to the floor behind your head. Keep your arms along your sides, with your palms facing down.

Plow Pose is said to be beneficial for the digestive and nervous systems, as well as reducing stress and anxiety. It's also said to be beneficial for people with insomnia and fatigue, as it helps to calm the mind and relax the body.

It's important to practice Plow Pose with a qualified teacher, as it can be difficult to perform correctly without proper guidance. Also, it's important to be mindful of the neck and spine, which can be easily strained if the pose is done incorrectly. It's not recommended for people with neck, back or shoulder injuries, or during pregnancy.

Prayer Pose

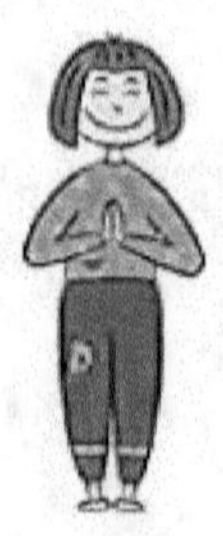

Prayer Pose

Prayer Pose, also known as Anjali Mudra or Namaste, is a common yoga pose that involves bringing the hands together in front of the heart in a prayer-like gesture. The pose can be performed standing or seated, and can be a starting or ending pose in a yoga practice. To come into the pose, begin by standing or sitting in a comfortable position. Bring the palms of your hands together in front of the heart, with the fingers pointing towards the sky. Press the palms together firmly and engage the triceps to create a sense of energy in the arms. Relax the shoulders away from the ears and keep the spine tall. Gently close the eyes and take a few deep breaths in and out through the nose. This pose can be used as a way to begin or end a yoga practice with a sense of gratitude and reverence.

Seated Twist Pose

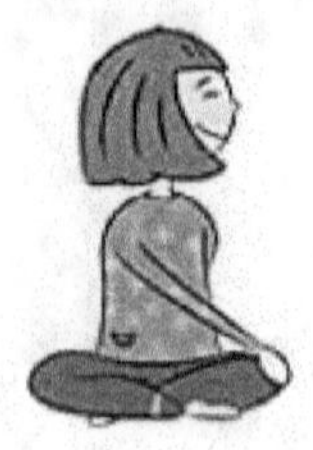

Seated Twist Pose

Seated Twist Pose, also known as Ardha Matsyendrasana, is a yoga pose that is considered to be an intermediate level pose. It is a seated twist that is said to be beneficial for the spine, shoulders, and hips, as well as for improving digestion and relieving stress.

To come into the pose, begin by sitting on the floor with your legs extended out in front of you. Bend your right knee and bring the right foot over the left knee, so that the right ankle is resting on the left knee. Keep the left leg extended and press the left foot firmly into the floor. Sit up tall and place your left hand behind your back, and your right hand on the outside of the right knee. Begin to twist your torso to the right, keeping your left shoulder pressing down, and look over the right shoulder. Hold for several breaths, then release and repeat on the other side.

It's important to keep the spine tall while doing this pose, and to twist from the base of the spine. You can use your hand on the knee to gently press down and deepen the twist. This pose is also good to do after a backbend and forward bend, as it helps to release tension on the spine.

It's important to be mindful of the spine, and if you have any back injuries or conditions, it's best to avoid this pose or to practice it with the guidance of a qualified yoga teacher.

Side Angle Pose

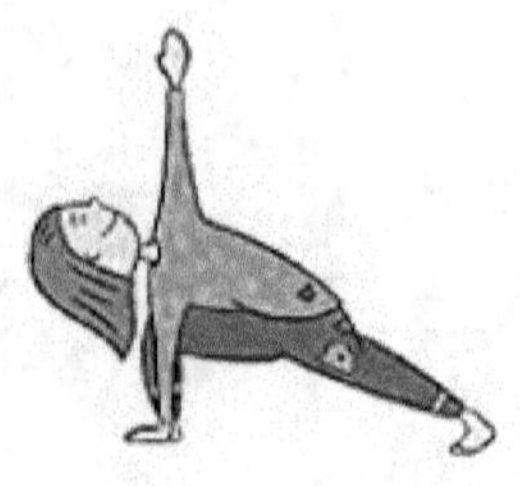

Side Angle Pose

Side Angle Pose, also known as Parsvakonasana, is a standing yoga pose that is known for strengthening the legs, core, and back, as well as stretching the hips, groins, and side body. It is considered an intermediate-level pose.

To come into the pose, begin by standing in Mountain Pose (Tadasana) with your feet together and your arms at your sides. Step your left foot back about 4-5 feet, and turn it out to a 90-degree angle. Turn your right foot out to a 90-degree angle as well, so that your hips are facing forward. Bend your right knee, making sure that your right knee is aligned over your right ankle. Bring your left hand to your left hip and extend your right arm up towards the ceiling. Keep your gaze forward and breathe deeply. Hold the pose for several breaths before switching sides.

It is a pose that improves balance, focus, and strengthens the legs, core, and back. It also opens the hips, groins, and side body, and is great for stretching the front of the body. It is a great pose to build strength and flexibility in the legs, hips and spine, it also helps to open up the chest and shoulders. The pose represents the balance and strength required to overcome difficult situations and encourages us to tap into our inner strength and determination.

It's important to keep the knee over the ankle and not to let it move forward past the toes, also to keep the back leg straight and engaged and to keep the tailbone down and engage the core. It's also important to keep the torso and both legs in a straight line with the front knee, and to stretch out of the side body, rather than collapsing in the front hip.

Staff Pose

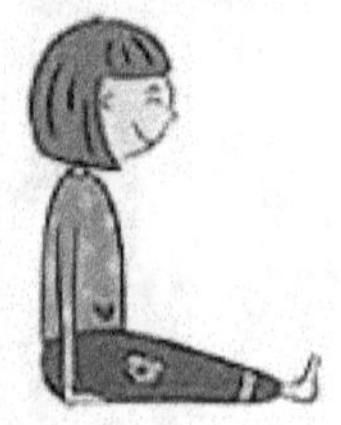

Staff Pose

Staff Pose, also known as Dandasana, is a seated
yoga pose that is considered to be a beginner level pose.
It is said to be beneficial for the spine, core, and legs,
as well as for improving posture and balance.

To come into the pose, begin by sitting on the floor with your legs
extended out in front of you. Sit up tall, with your spine straight
and your shoulders relaxed. Place your hands on the floor next
to your hips, with your fingers pointing forward. Press your
sitting bones into the floor, and engage your core muscles to keep
your spine straight. Gaze forward and keep your breath steady.

It's important to keep the spine tall and to engage the thigh muscles
to protect the knee joints. You can use a block or cushion to sit on
if your hips are not able to touch the floor comfortably. It's also

important to come out of the pose slowly and with mindful movements.

Staff pose is considered to be a very beneficial pose for the spine, core and leg muscles. It's also a good pose for those who spend a lot of time sitting, as it helps to stretch out the spine and core muscles. It's also a good pose to practice before seated forward bends, as it helps to prepare the body. Additionally, it helps to improve posture and balance, and also helps to release tension in the lower back.

Tree Pose

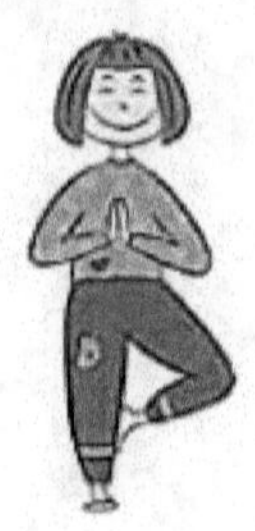# Tree Pose

Tree Pose, also known as Vrikshasana, is a standing balance pose in yoga. It is considered a beginner-intermediate level pose and is known for helping to improve balance and stability. To come into the pose, begin by standing in Mountain Pose (Tadasana) with your feet together and your hands at your sides. Shift your weight to your left foot and bend your right knee, lifting your right foot off the ground. Place the sole of your right foot on the inside of your left thigh, with the heel as close to the hip as possible. Keep the foot flexed and engage the thigh and calf muscles to maintain balance. Bring your hands together at the heart center in prayer position, or raise them above your head, palms touching or fingers interlaced. Keep the gaze forward, and breathe deeply. Hold the pose for several breaths, then release and repeat on the opposite side.

Warrior 1 Pose

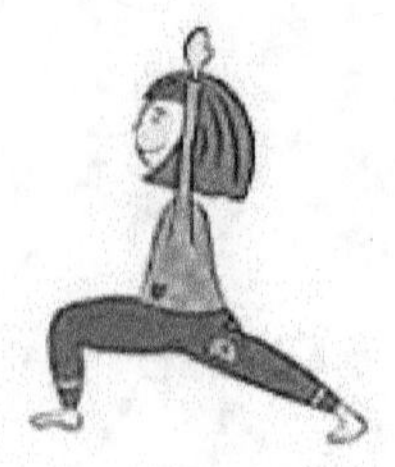

Warrior 1 Pose

Warrior 1 Pose, also known as Virabhadrasana I, is a standing yoga pose that is known for strengthening the legs, arms, and core, as well as opening the hips and chest. It is considered an intermediate-level pose.

To come into the pose, begin by standing in Mountain Pose (Tadasana) with your feet together and your arms at your sides. Step your left foot back about 4-5 feet, and turn it out to a 90-degree angle. Bend your right knee, making sure that your right knee is aligned over your right ankle. Bring your arms up over your head, with the palms facing each other, reaching towards the sky. Keep your gaze forward and breathe deeply. Hold the pose for several breaths before switching sides.

It is a powerful pose that improves balance, focus, and

strengthens the legs, arms, and core. It also opens the hips and chest, and is great for stretching the front of the body. It is a warrior pose, representing the strength and power that lies within each of us, and encourages the practitioner to tap into their inner strength and confidence.

Warrior 2 Pose

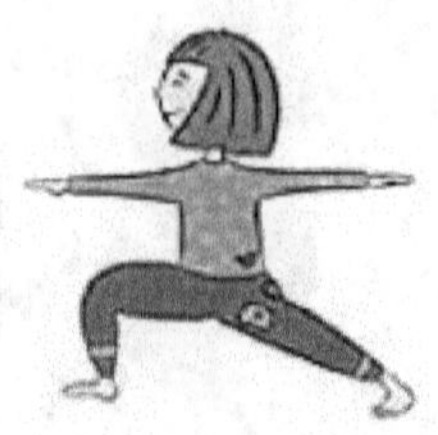

Warrior 2 Pose

Warrior 2 Pose, also known as Virabhadrasana II, is a standing yoga pose that is known for strengthening the legs, arms, and core, as well as stretching the hips, groins and chest. It is considered an intermediate-level pose.

To come into the pose, begin by standing in Mountain Pose (Tadasana) with your feet together and your arms at your sides. Step your left foot back about 4-5 feet, and turn it out to a 90-degree angle. Turn your right foot out to a 90-degree angle as well, so that your hips are facing forward. Bend your right knee, making sure that your right knee is aligned over your right ankle. Bring your arms out to the sides, parallel with the floor, with the left arm facing forward and the right arm facing backward. Your gaze should be over the front hand. Hold the pose for several breaths before switching sides.

It is a powerful pose that improves balance, focus, and strengthens the legs, arms, and core. It also opens the hips, groins and chest, and is great for stretching the front of the body. It is a warrior pose, representing the strength and power that lies within each of us, and encourages the practitioner to tap into their inner strength and confidence. It also helps to improve endurance and stamina.

It's important to keep the knee over the ankle and not to let it move forward past the toes, also to keep the back leg straight and engaged and to keep the tailbone down and engage the core.

Warrior 3 Pose

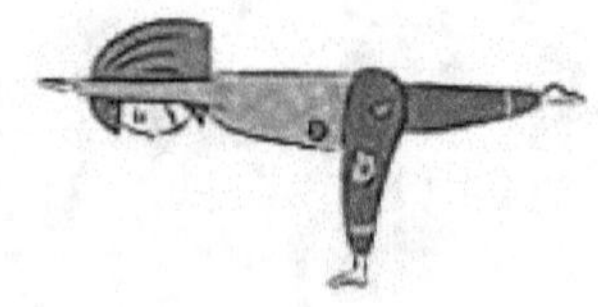

Warrior 3 Pose

Warrior 3 Pose, also known as Virabhadrasana III, is a standing yoga pose that is known for strengthening the legs, core, and back, as well as improving balance and focus. It is considered an advanced-level pose.

To come into the pose, begin by standing in Mountain Pose (Tadasana) with your feet together and your arms at your sides. Shift your weight onto your left foot and lift your right foot off the ground. Slowly begin to lean forward, hinging at the hips, as you raise your right leg behind you, keeping it straight and parallel to the ground. Keep your gaze forward and extend both arms out in front of you. As you reach a point of balance, you may choose to lower your right hand to touch the floor or a block, while keeping your left arm extended forward. Hold the pose for several breaths before switching sides.

It is a challenging pose that requires a strong core, leg and back muscles, and balance, and it's a great way to improve your balance and focus, as well as strengthen the legs, core and back. It also helps to open the chest and stretch the shoulders, hips, and hamstrings. The pose represents the balance and strength required to overcome difficult situations and encourages us to tap into our inner strength and determination.

It's important to keep the lifted leg and extended arm parallel to the ground, engage your core and keep your gaze forward. To help with balance, it's recommended to practice it near a wall or use a chair for support.

www.ingramcontent.com/pod-product-compliance
Lightning Source LLC
Chambersburg PA
CBHW061048250726
48653CB00001B/305